CW00557634

THE OLDER P
CONSENT AN

Report of the
British Medical Association
and the
Royal College of Nursing

Published by the British Medical Association
Tavistock Square, London WC1H 9JP
April 1995

THE OLDER PERSON: CONSENT AND CARE
Report of the
British Medical Association
and the
Royal College of Nursing

Unless we are old already, then the next "old people" will be us. No pill or regimen known or likely, could transform the latter years of life as fully as could a change in our vision of age and a militancy in achieving that change.

Alex Comfort, A Good Age, 1977

First published in 1995

British Library Cataloguing Publication Data
A catalogue record for this book is available from the British Library

ISBN 0 7279 0912 6

Typeset in Great Britain by Apek Typesetters Ltd., Nailsea, Bristol.
Printed and bound by Derrys

Contents

Membership of the Steering Group

Professor Christine Chapman	Emeritus Professor of Nursing Member, BMA Medical Ethics Committee
Mr Stuart Darby	Royal College of Nursing
Dr Fleur Fisher	Head of Ethics, Science and Information Division, BMA
Ms Hazel Heath	Royal College of Nursing
Dr J Anthony Hicklin	Consultant Rheumatologist Member, BMA Medical Ethics Committee
Dr J Stuart Horner (ex officio)	Director of Public Health Chairman, BMA Medical Ethics Committee
Dr Vincent Leach	General Practitioner Member, BMA Medical Ethics Committee
Dr Steven Luttrell	Senior Registrar in Medicine for the Elderly Whittington Hospital NHS Trust
Mr Jim Marr	Royal College of Nursing
Ms Evelyn McEwen	Divisional Director, Age Concern England
Ms Lynne Phair	Royal College of Nursing
Dr Anne Rodway	General Practitioner Deputy Chairman, BMA Medical Ethics Committee
Dr Kevin Somerville	Consultant Physician St Bartholomew's Hospital, London
Ms Ann Sommerville	Advisor to the BMA on medical ethics
Ms Henrietta Wallace	Senior Research Officer BMA Ethics, Audit and Careers Department
Written by	Henrietta Wallace
Contributors	Stuart Darby
	Hazel Heath
	Steven Luttrell
	Ann Sommerville
Editors	Amy Salter
	Dawn Waterman
Editorial Secretariat	Gillian Romano
Project Manager	Rosemary Weston

British Medical Association, BMA House, Tavistock Square,
London WC1H 9JP.   Telephone 0171 383 6286

Chapter 1
The Problem of
Consent and Care

Frederick Clark was uncertain of his future. Never in his eighty-four years had he been faced with this sort of decision. Staff at the residential home where Mr Clark lived were concerned that his increasing tendency to wander would lead to an accident on the busy road outside. They suggested Mr Clark be relocated to another home in a less busy area. His doctor suggested medication that would decrease his tendency to wander and would also decrease the frequency of his memory lapses. Mr Clark's daughter and son-in-law were not happy with either of these proposals and suggested that nothing be changed. Yet, Mr Clark knew something had to be done. He knew his memory lapses were becoming more frequent. He knew he would sometimes find himself near the busy road outside the home, but have no idea how he had arrived there. Despite his failing health and uncertain future, however, Mr Clark's greatest fear was that a decision about his future would be made without his input. Could the residential home, the doctors and his daughter make a decision without consulting him? Did they really know that he had periods of lucidity and that he had definite preferences about this decision? What would he, could he, do if he was unhappy with the circumstances which were 'decided' for him?

Frederick Clark could be any one of us in our later years. He is indeed one of the growing number of older people facing similar dilemmas today. Mr Clark's case illustrates one of the many ethical problems concerning consent and care faced daily by older people and those who care for them.

The British Medical Association and the Royal College of Nursing are aware of concerns about the treatment of older people and the provision of care for this section of our population. In this report, we focus mainly on the ethical problems which arise daily for the minority of older people who require care and treatment, particularly problems related to consent, and our ethical and legal duties as professionals towards these people.

Older people have the same rights to services, and to health care in particular, as do other members of society. We know that the life of an older person is just as valuable as that of a younger individual and judgements about the quality of that life are the sole prerogative of the person living it. We know there is no justification for dismissing these people as a burden, or for judging the value of life solely on the basis of age. Yet, despite these facts, the rights of older people are often ignored, and the ability of these people to dictate the quality of their life is often overlooked by well-intentioned individuals. Most older people are capable of caring for themselves. This report focuses on the small proportion of older individuals who:

- need help to carry on their lives with some degree of independence
- are cognitively impaired and are therefore unable to consent to treatment
- are capable of giving consent to treatment, but whose wishes may be overlooked
- have difficulty communicating their wishes.

1:1　What is the purpose of this report?

The realities of providing good quality, day-to-day care, especially for people in an institutional setting and with varying degrees of mental impairment, rarely sit easily within the framework of patient rights which we acknowledge to be the ideal. In some cases, provision of care would grind to a halt if requirements for unpressured and informed patient consent were observed as fully as some textbooks advocate. The concepts of **partnership**, **interdependence**, and **mutual respect** are more helpful than strict adherence to principles of autonomy. The purpose of this report, therefore, is to provide general guidance about how we can address the gaps between the theory and practical reality of care.

This report has been prepared by specialists in the care of older people from the British Medical Association, the Royal College of Nursing, Age Concern and other experts. It is written for all those caring for older people; medical and nursing staff, other health professionals, non-professional care staff, lawyers, social service personnel, and family members. It is designed to be a *working* document that provides background information to the issues, as well as practical guidance that you can refer to quickly, on a daily basis.

Case studies are presented throughout this document to illustrate good practice regarding consent and care.

1:2 Who is the older person?

As people in the developed world live longer and fitter lives, perceptions of "old age" change. Regrettably, the attitudes perpetuated portray the increasing population of older people as a social problem or as a demographic disaster[1] rather than as a positive asset. The majority of older people enjoy good health and contribute to society in many ways. Frailty and the need to be cared for by others is characteristic only of a minority of people towards the end of their lives. Although this report focuses on this group, much of our discussion is also applicable to other patients. We recognise that there are risks in singling out any group since this may lead to a failure to perceive them as individuals.

1:2.1 The facts

- **A person's risk of receiving inadequate health care increases with his or her age.** Much of the debate about prioritising health resources in this country has centred around allegations of "rationing by age" and not by individual need and ability to benefit, despite the rejection of such blanket decision-making by health professionals.

- **Older people are often marginalised according to economic or administrative definitions of population which concentrate on the relative proportions of people in paid employment and those who are not.** The standard

3

retirement age of 65 for men is regarded as the beginning of "old age" even though many people (including most women at present) retire earlier and some professional or skilled workers continue in paid employment beyond 65. Sociological changes, such as the increasing numbers of unemployed younger people in many western countries, mean that "retirement" or "pensionable age" has diminished in importance for many people.

- **People in their mid-60s have relatively the same level of physical fitness, mental agility and service needs as people of pre-retirement age.** Some of these people are themselves dealing successfully with the care and management of older relatives.

- **Most older people need only minimal help with the self-care and domestic tasks required to maintain independence; often these are tasks that other age groups also find problematic.** Ageing is not inevitably accompanied by dependence and frailty. However, the need for assistance in performing activities of daily living increases with increasing age. It is estimated that 15% of people over 65 need help with some tasks they previously performed independently[2] but for most the degree of assistance required is relatively small. McGlone[3] estimated, for example, that only 4% of people aged 65-69 were unable to wash themselves but 16% of the same age group had trouble cutting their toe-nails. At age 85+, 31% needed help with washing and 65% could not cut their toe-nails. Toe-nail cutting and heavy domestic work are two activities which seem most troublesome for a large number of older people but only very small proportions are unable to perform essential tasks, such as household management or cooking for themselves.

- **Only 7% of disabled people aged 65-69 live in communal establishments.** Most live in private households, although predictably the proportion living in institutions increases with age.[4]

1:2.2 Their needs
These facts do not minimise the problems regarding the provision of services for older people. The section of the older

population addressed in this report have particular health care needs, or require more than basic assistance, as illustrated below:

- 16% of people over 65 cannot do their own shopping; the actual number of people comprising this 16% is about 1.4 million.

- It is estimated that one in five people aged 85+ will have dementia[5] and three in five will have a long-standing illness which limits their activity.[6] Conditions such as heart problems, arthritis, sight or hearing defects, or incontinence make some aspects of daily living an effort, especially if they are exacerbated by the limitations of poor housing, low income or poor public transport.

- Mental health problems occur at all ages, but there is a cumulative effect apparent in higher levels of mental illness in older people. It is sometimes said that "depression is the epidemic condition of old age"[7] but such statements are complicated by problems of definition and study methodology.

- Negative societal attitudes and reluctance to devote greater resources to a variety of issues which particularly affect older people may contribute to how their difficulties are perceived.

1:3 What are the specific problems of consent and care?

Every day, health professionals encounter numerous decisions regarding consent to the treatment and care of older people. It is vital that all carers are fully informed of their legal and ethical obligations, as well as of the rights of the people they treat. The following statements briefly outline the issues and problems carers should consider.

- **Health professionals work according to established ethical codes which apply to all the people they care for.** The same standards of care and degree of respect apply to all. The same ethical issues of patient confidentiality and the need for consent apply. Well intentioned procedures, without the valid consent of the person to accept it or refuse it, are not acceptable.

- **The care of older people requires more than the services of doctors and nurses.** Successful management of daily problems is likely to involve professionals and non-professionals, relatives, neighbours, social work teams and voluntary organisations. This makes concepts of confidentiality harder to define. Similarly, "care" is broader than simply managing people's physical or mental problems. Health professionals and carers may have to become involved in looking at aspects of patients' lifestyle, financial arrangements, domestic situation, familial relationships and personal hygiene.

- **Marginalisation of any section of the community is due to a variety of factors which are mostly beyond the influence of health professionals.** The type of care older people need may be affected by the availability of adequate heating and nutrition outside the care setting, as well as the existence of supportive family or social ties. Adequate pension arrangements, provision of long-stay hospital or nursing home beds, residential home places or sheltered housing, good public transport and accessibility to shops and services all affect health, and require considerable forethought on society's part.

- **It may be difficult to judge what a person wants, if his or her body or mind is failing.** If a person is unable to express his or her opinions, or retain information long enough to make a decision, there may be difficulties in judging what this person would want, bearing in mind their former views and values.

- **Older people are more likely than most other adults to experience an erosion of their rights.** The concept of patient and elderly "empowerment" is said to have grown partly because rights are respected within society only if claimed personally or through a proxy.[8] The ability to be heard and to exercise control over one's life contributes to positive health outcomes.[9] A key step to empowerment in health care is the legal requirement of valid patient consent. Increasing interest in mechanisms, such as advance statements, or medical treatment attorneys bear witness to the notion of self-expression by older people regarding health care decisions. Power in decision making, however, depends on knowledge and an ability to exercise choice. Therefore, one of the issues we consider arises from the duties of health professionals to provide information in an accessible manner and to enhance patient capacity when this is achievable. (See BMA and Law Society guidance on assessment of mental capacity).

- **People who are perceived, or who perceive themselves, as dependent upon the services of others may experience difficulty in asserting their rights.** People who have been resident in institutions or other places where decisions are often made for them may acquire the habit of acquiescence or become accustomed to coercion. Some ethical and caring institutions would find it impossible in practice to provide good standards of care if individuals were not encouraged to conform in certain matters. The problem for the health professional is to ensure that concerns for individual and group welfare do not overshadow individual rights and that people who may not be accustomed to making decisions are encouraged to have a voice in those matters which affect them.

- **Do not resuscitate orders** must always be made on an individual basis. The Royal College of Nursing and the British Medical Association agree that it is unacceptable for institutions to have a policy preventing resuscitation teams from treating certain groups of patients.

Each of these issues is addressed in chapters 2–5. Suggestions and recommendations are presented in boldface type, followed by a discussion of the issue and illustrative case studies. A summary of the conclusions and recommendations is presented in chapter 6.

1 Bond J, Coleman P, Pearce S. 1993. "Ageing in the Twentieth Century". In Bond J, Coleman P, Peace S (eds) *Ageing in Society: an introduction to social gerontology*. London: Sage Publications

2 Office of Population and Census Surveys. 1985. *Inability to Undertake Mobility, Self-Care and Domestic Tasks in the Population 65+*. London: OPCS.

3 McGlone F. 1992. Disability and Dependency in Old Age: A Demographic and Social Audit. Family Policy Studies Centre, London.

4 Johnson M. 1993. Dependency and Interdependency. In *Ageing in Society: an introduction to social gerontology*. London: Sage Publications.

5 Kay DW. 1991. Psychiatry of old age. The epidemiology of dementia: a review of recent work. *Reviews in Clinical Gerontology*.

6 Department of Health. 1992. The Health of Elderly People. An Epidemiological Overview. HMSO, London.

7 Johnson M. 1993. Dependency and Interdependency. In *Ageing in Society an introduction to social gerontology*. London: Sage Publications.

8 Clark P. 1987. Individual Autonomy, Cooperative Empowerment and Planning for Long-Term Care Decision Making. *Journal of Ageing Studies* 1:65.

9 Rodin J. 1986. Ageing and Health: effects on the sense of control. *Science* 233: 1271.

Chapter 2
Consent and Care in Day-to-Day Situations

In the day-to-day reality of working with older people, many situations arise in which older individuals, to varying degrees, may be unable to understand or to make or express choices. These situations can occur in any setting, and may be temporary or ongoing. The inability of the older person may be caused by mental or physical incapacity. Wherever or however these situations occur, they raise dilemmas for the health professionals involved.

In many daily decisions the appropriate path of action is not clear. **Very few people are totally incapable of making any decision.** For example, it could be assumed that a person with advanced dementia was unable to select his or her own clothes. In reality, given a rail of clothes from which to select, the individual will often be able to make a choice.

> Following a cerebral vascular accident, Mr Thomas appeared confused and unable to make decisions. It was assumed he was unable to select what he would wear each morning. In reality, however, Mr Thomas was able to communicate his choice if he was offered adequate time and appropriate methods of communication which acknowledged his difficulties.

The older person may well be making decisions on daily activities (eg, personal hygiene, eating, walking or clothing), on receiving care, treatment or investigations (eg, medications or wound care) or on housing or finance.

2:1 Promoting patient autonomy

Current medical and nursing literature advocates a caring model based on an equal, open, mutually respectful partnership. It focuses on the right of each patient to make decisions about his or her life and to be responsible for the consequences. The model emphasises the individual's values, choices, autonomy and freedom from controlling intervention. The responsibility of the health professional is to respect the individual patient's values and rights and to facilitate this person's self-determination, even if the patient's values conflict with those of the other party. This relationship is described as the Patient Autonomy Model.

2:1.1 Difficulties in promoting patient autonomy

Not all patients are capable of acting autonomously. The person's *capacity* to make decisions may change according to the environment, the people around him or her, the time of day, physiological changes or medication reactions. A person's competence to make decisions can therefore be difficult to establish. Partial capacity is not the same as capacity or incapacity. Competence in these situations is therefore a relative, rather than an absolute, state.

In situations where a patient is deemed to be incapable of making a decision at that particular time, professionals may make decisions based on what is in the best interests of the patient. When nurses have established a relationship with a patient they may assume that, because they understand the patient's values, they can predict what sort of decisions the patient might make in the circumstances. Although these kinds of professional decisions may be appropriate, health professionals should be careful about making any assumptions about the patient's wishes and the following considerations should be acknowledged before action is taken.

- Particular difficulties arise when the patient has mental impairment. These people are human beings whose rights and autonomous choices should be preserved. Yet, they also are vulnerable and in need of protection, support and care. Dilemmas are inevitable in this situation.

- Health professionals have their own perspectives based on knowledge and experience. They also have values and beliefs about, for example, quality of life, death, health and the utility of specific treatments. Professionals often perceive situations differently from a patient. Indeed, patients' mental competence may be questioned for the first time when they do not comply with care or treatment advice. It can be difficult to control professional biases.

- Many different professionals may be working with each patient and this can bring many different sets of values and beliefs into the decision-making process. The patient's carers may similarly bring their own values, thus adding a further dimension.

- The relationship between the professional and the older patient, particularly a person with mental impairment, is not an equal balance of power. Therefore, the older person may comply without questioning.

2:2   Assessing the older person's capacity to make decisions

Situations may arise in which an older person refuses treatment (for example, medication) or care (for example, to be helped to walk, eat or wash). In these instances, professionals must ask themselves, Is the refusal to allow care or treatment a manifestation of the underlying organic illness in part or in whole? An acute confusional state is a frequent presentation of many disease processes in old people and may produce denial, or forceful warding off of efforts to care for, investigate and treat. The distinction between coherent refusal and delirium or confusion can usually be made on clinical grounds, but may require expert psychiatric opinion.

The relationship between the professional and the older person needs to be dynamic and each situation must be assessed individually. A person's capacity to make decisions can be conceptualised as being based along a continuum (see Figure 1). At one end are people who are fully able to understand, make and express choices; at the other end are people who are deemed to have no decisional capabilities. The majority of people are somewhere between these two points, but the exact position may vary from one occasion to another.

Total independence and ability to understand, make and express choices	Profound inability to understand, make and express choices
Autonomy Model	Beneficence of Paternalism Models

Figure 1

If a decision is to be made about the treatment of a 'competent' older patient, this should be discussed in broad terms with the older person and, provided the older person consents, also with a relative or friend. Many dependent patients, who have the capacity to make certain decisions will, nevertheless, choose to let another make the decisions on their behalf. It is important to ask such patients about this and to ensure they are not forced to make decisions which they would find onerous, or which would cause them anxiety.

2:2.1 Maximising the older person's capacity to make decisions

There are several ways health professionals can help to maximise the older person's autonomy in decision-making:

- assess the capacity to make decisions on a decision-specific basis and do not make assumptions about competence before adequate assessment
- appreciate that incompetence in one area of decision-making does not necessarily mean incompetence in another
- delay decision-making until an opportunity presents itself, for example a lucid phase
- allow time for the person to make decisions
- written information about the risks and benefits of treatment can help overcome poor memory, allow people to review and reinforce what they have been told and to reflect on the issues in their own time
- work to understand the individual's values and how the person would wish to live; this understanding can arise from

11

understanding an individual's biography and values, and may also arise from the day-to-day relationship

- do not assume that the older person's values are the same as your values
- emphasise functioning rather than diagnosis
- permit the person to choose and *facilitate* that choice
- avoid transferring decision-making to relatives when the patient has not been included in the process.

2:3 Making choices for the older person

2:3.1 *Choices in daily activities*

Some of the most difficult day-to-day dilemmas arise when an older person with cognitive impairment makes a choice that the professionals believe he or she would *not* make if he or she were not cognitively impaired. For example, Mr Peters, a man with dementia, defecates into his pants and refuses to remove them.

In such situations, nurses usually assume that, were he not mentally impaired, Mr Peters would not wish to walk around with faeces in his pants. They then use various techniques to encourage him to remove his pants and to wash or bath.

Although the nurses make some assumptions about the patient's values (ie, cleanliness) in these situations, they also consider what would be less degrading and less damaging for him. In working to minimise the damage and degradation they utilise a range of techniques.

- reinforcing successes, not failures (ie, not emphasising that Mr Peters has defecated)
- preventing failures whenever possible (eg, encouraging patients to go to the lavatory before they need to go)
- limiting the choices so that the person does not fail (eg, presenting choices of appropriate clothing for the weather, or appropriate food for the time of day)
- guiding the choices (eg, rather than inviting Mr Peters to bathe, saying "I've run a bath for you").

Nurses also use a range of skills, particularly in relationship-building, communicating and supporting. If the patient refuses (eg, the bath), they may divert his attention or repeat the request once he has forgotten the original conversation. Nurses also try to maintain maximum autonomy for the patient by facilitating choices in as many aspects of daily life as possible; for example, what time to get up, what to eat, what to wear. This is particularly important when circumstances have led to a diminution in the skills of competent decision-making (for example, if the person has become institutionalised). Advocates also can help to promote the views of the older person. Currently, many advocacy schemes are developing across the country (see Chapter 4).

2:3.2 Making significant decisions

The point at which acceptable risk becomes unacceptable can be determined only in individual circumstances. Situations in which people with mental impairment are making decisions about their futures raise particular dilemmas for health professionals. For example, Joan Richards, an 82-year-old woman with dementia, insisted on remaining within her own home. When at home, she was content, but did not consider eating or drinking. The professionals involved wanted to support her choice and developed a package of care in which a community psychiatric nurse and a care assistant visited Miss Richards at prescribed times of day. They prepared food and drink for her and the nurse monitored her health.

Despite her dementia, Miss Richards' autonomy had been preserved. However, the professionals received the criticism that they had placed her at risk. In these circumstances, by widening the boundaries of what they define as acceptable risk, professionals face increased discomfort concerning their accountability.

One factor that may tip the balance of a situation from acceptable to unacceptable is when an individual places other members of the community at risk. In these circumstances, ethical concern for the safety, health and welfare of the community may enforce a decision in which the needs of the community take precedence over those of an individual.

If we regard older people as *individuals* with their own life histories, values and contributions, we are more likely to promote and facilitate the autonomy of the older person, whatever the circumstances.

Chapter 3
General Ethical
Principles of Consent

The relationship between health professionals and patients is based on the concept of **partnership**. Ideally, decisions are made through frank discussion, in which the carer's expertise and the patient's needs and preferences are shared. The patient's consent to being examined and to receiving treatment is the trigger which allows the interchange to take place. Treatment is undertaken only as a result of patients being actively involved in deciding what is to be done to them.

3:1   Definition of Consent

Before a person can be given treatment, his or her valid consent is required, except where the law provides the authority to treat patients without consent (see section 3:3).

Consent is defined broadly as the "voluntary and continuing permission of the patient to receive a particular treatment, based on adequate knowledge of the purpose, nature, likely effects and risks of that treatment including the likelihood of its success and any alternatives to it. Permission given under any unfair or undue pressure is not consent".[10]

3:2   Assessing a Patient's Capacity to Consent

It is the personal responsibility of any health professional proposing to treat a patient, to determine whether the patient has the capacity to give a valid consent. Assessing a patient's capacity to make a decision about his or her medical treatment is a matter for clinical judgement, guided by current professional practice and subject to legal requirements. The BMA and the Law Society have produced guidance on the assessment of mental capacity.

In order to have *capacity*, the patient must be able to:

- understand, in broad terms and simple language, what the medical treatment is, its purpose and nature, and why the treatment is being proposed for them
- understand its principal benefits, risks and alternatives
- understand, in broad terms, the consequences of not receiving the proposed treatment
- possess the capacity to make a free choice (ie, free from pressure)
- retain the information long enough for an effective decision.

3:2.1 *Ways to determine an older person's capacity to consent:*

Invite the patient to ask questions and answer the questions fully, frankly and truthfully in language the patient understands. Occasionally, there may be a compelling reason, in the patient's interest, for not disclosing certain information, but this should be an exceptional situation. For example, in cases where the person will not be able to remember the content of the conversation, but will live with the emotions that are left by it, it can be beneficial not to give information to patients. This is also true for people who have lost the ability to reason, and who are unable to debate and negotiate with you. Any additional information imparted to the patient is a matter of judgement for the health professional proposing the treatment.

Mrs Leeds has very poor short-term memory and becomes agitated and at risk when she goes outside her residential home. Today, she wants to leave the residential unit to do some shopping.

If the professional spends time explaining to her that she is not physically or mentally able to do the shopping, it may cause Mrs Leeds great distress by giving her a momentary insight into her health status.

It may be appropriate to divert Mrs Leeds' attention by guiding her back upstairs to have a drink, breaking her concentration, and removing thoughts of wanting to leave from her head. While not condoning lying, it is sometimes more therapeutic to withhold the true facts in order to reduce stress.

Use your professional judgement to decide *when* it is appropriate to give patients news which may be harmful to them. The following case study illustrates this.

Two sisters in their eighties were assaulted at home. One died immediately of her injuries. The surviving sister, who was also badly injured, asked after her sister.

It was felt that informing her of the death of her sister at that time would be deleterious to her recovery. Instead, she was told later, when her situation had improved and she was better able to cope with the news.

Give information not only *prior to* seeking a patient's consent, but also *during* a particular course of treatment, so that the patient can decide whether to request that treatment be altered or stopped, according to his or her needs and desires. Patients should be told that their consent to treatment can be withdrawn at any time and that fresh consent is required before further treatment can be given or reinstated. If they choose, patients can designate a named person to make decisions; the patients can simply state the outcome they want without having to decide the process by which it is achieved.

Recognise when the patient has received enough information or does not want to know certain information. This is a difficult business, but health professionals should detect both verbal and non verbal cues from the patient about how much the patient wants to know. It is very important to listen to the older person and to give him or her ample time to decide. Health professionals should make it clear that their door is always open for further discussion. Some older people are keen to know the outcome of the treatment (eg, how well they will be able to walk) but do not want to know the details of the treatment (eg, how a hip replacement is done) People have a right *not* to know information about themselves that they do not feel ready to hear. Yet, health professionals should not assume that a patient does not want to know all the details of the treatment, simply because the health professional finds it difficult to give the information to the patient.

Encourage, but do not force, patients to make difficult choices. In most cases, people will be prepared to make choices, but occasionally the patient's final choice is to let the health professional decide. This is not a denial of choice and the patient who makes a decision regarding one aspect of treatment should not be seen as relinquishing choice on other issues. If given appropriate support, patients may feel able to deal with very difficult choices despite their anxieties.

Eighty-three-year-old Mr Davidson was diagnosed with a life-threatening condition. The clinician was unsure from Mr Davidson's comments whether he wished to know the full implications of the diagnosis. Following further discussion, and using both verbal and non verbal cues, Mr Davidson made clear that he did not want to know the diagnosis until after the New Year, so that he and his family could enjoy Christmas without the knowledge of his impending death. The clinician felt that Mr Davidson instinctively knew the news would be bad, but did not want it made explicit before the holidays.

3:3 Treating people who have the capacity to consent, when consent is not given

Ordinarily, a person capable of giving consent can only be given medical treatment for a mental disorder against his or her wishes, in accordance with the provisions of Part IV of the Mental Health Act 1983. These are mirrored in the 1984 Mental Health (Scotland) Act and the 1986 Mental Health (Northern Ireland) Order. On rare occasions involving emergencies, where it is not immediately possible to apply the provisions of the Mental Health Act, a patient suffering from a mental disorder which is leading to behaviour that is an immediate serious danger to him or herself, or to other people, may be given the minimum treatment necessary to avert danger. It must be emphasised that the administration of such treatment is not an alternative to giving treatment under the Mental Health Act, nor should its administration delay the proper application of the Act to the patient at the earliest opportunity.

3:4 Treating people who have impaired capacity

As a general principle, encourage patients to exercise their decision-making capacity to its limits. The fact that a

17

person acts in a way that an ordinary, prudent person would not act, is not in itself evidence of impaired capacity. The capacity to consent in a valid way may be affected by many factors, including pain or fatigue. In addition, some patients suffer from mental disorder or impairment. None of these conditions necessarily prevent the patient from giving valid consent. A wide spectrum of ability is found within the group of patients whose competence to decide is permanently or temporarily affected. Competency may also vary over time and health professionals may need to be more selective about timing in order to raise the issues with the patient in a meaningful way. Pending legislation based on the English Law Commission's review of measures for making decisions for people who cannot decide for themselves, the British Medical Association issued interim guidelines for the medical profession on the treatment of such patients. These are available from the BMA's Ethics Division.

Katherine Jones is 79 years old and suffers from a dementing illness, including short-term memory problems, as well as delusions that her husband is having an affair, that there are children in her bed, and that her mother is in the flat. Occasionally, she claims that her husband has beaten her, but there is no evidence to support this. Mrs Jones has lucid moments, but quickly slips back into her muddled state. She is very anxious and distressed by her beliefs, as she has been married for 54 happy years. Her husband is her main carer and is also distressed.

Stelazine is prescribed. Mrs Jones is unable to retain any information about the drug, or to understand why she needs it. But she does remember that she is very upset and worried and that she does not want to feel this way. In order to preserve her relationship with her husband, and to ensure no deterioration in her condition, it is felt to be in Mrs Jones' best interests to prescribe the medication even though her capacity to consent is impaired. The medication will enhance her autonomy and give back her peace of mind.

3:5 Treating people who do not have the capacity to consent

If an adult patient is not able to give consent, either through temporary loss of consciousness or continuing mental incapacity, health professionals must act in the

patient's best interests.[11] There is no clear test for determining what course of action will be in a person's best interests but a health professional will want to consult with others in the team caring for the patient in order to reach a decision. In law, no person can give consent to treatment on behalf of another adult. The Law Commission is currently exploring possibilities for changing this law. However, if treatment is necessary to safeguard the life, health or well-being of the patient, then health professionals are not only entitled, but may be legally bound, to give treatment without consent. When a patient is only temporarily incompetent, treatment which can reasonably be postponed should not be given until the patient regains competency.

Elective treatments, such as health screening or preventive measures, should be offered if it is in the patient's best interests, while taking into account the invasiveness of the elective measure. If mentally incapacitated patients do not overtly object to a particular measure, then they should not be deprived of its benefits.

Remember that in some circumstances treatment may not necessarily be the best course of action for the patient. For example, in the case of a terminally ill patient, it may not be in his or her best interests to be given emergency life saving treatment if it will only prolong life for a short time. In each case, therefore, it must be the patient's best interests which govern the extent of treatment.

Treatment should not be given where there is convincing evidence that the patient would have withheld consent. Such evidence may take the form of an advance statement which addresses the particular situation which has arisen (see section 3:11). For more detailed information about advance statements, see the BMA's code of practice for health professionals on advance statements.

3:6 Consent and the Mental Health Act 1983

Patients who lack the capacity to give consent may be admitted to hospital under the Mental Health Act 1983 if they fall within the remit of the relevant section. Thus under section 2, a patient may be admitted for assessment if "he is

19

suffering from a mental disorder of a nature or degree which warrants the detention of the patient in a hospital for at least a limited period" and "he ought to be so detained in the interests of his own health or safety or with a view to the protection of others". Under section 3, a patient may be admitted for treatment if "he is suffering from mental illness" and "it is necessary for the health or safety of the patient or for the protection of other persons that he receive such treatment and it cannot be provided unless he is detained under this section". Treatment under the Mental Health Act is confined to the treatment of mental disorder.

According to section 1 of the Act a mental disorder means, among other things, mental illness. Although mental illness is not defined in the Act, the case of W v L (1974) QB 711 makes it clear that it should be given its ordinary meaning. Thus the sections can be applied to patients with dementia and arguably for patients with acute confusional states.

As a matter of practice, however, doctors rarely use the Mental Health Act for patients with dementia or acute confusion, as it is often felt that the use of the Act will cause a further burden of emotional stress to families and carers. The admission and treatment of such patients will usually be by way of the common law principles of "necessity" or "the patient's best interests".

3:7 Consulting people close to the patient

The consent of relatives to treat an incapacitated patient is not recognised in law; however, relatives should be involved in decisions about the patient's treatment whenever possible. As no person can give consent to treatment on behalf of another adult, it is useless to ask relatives to sign consent forms for the treatment of adult incapacitated patients. Nevertheless, those close to the patient can play an important role in the decision-making process and may also be helpful in supplying information about the social background of the patient. However, the views of those close to the patient should only be taken into account when it is clear that these people have the patient's welfare closely at heart and may be able to reflect the patient's known preferences in circumstances when the patient cannot express these.

If the patient has previously been autonomous, decisions

should be based on the patient's known views and preferences. People close to the patient may be able to indicate what these preferences are. Treatment which is contrary to the known wishes of the patient when competent, is rarely justified. However, in rare circumstances, overriding a patient's previously expressed wishes may be justifiable.

The Law Commission has proposed introducing legislation which would give health professionals legal authority to treat a person who is not able to consent, subject to certain limitations, if it would be in the patient's best interests to do so. This is currently the case at common law, following the case of *Re F* [1990] 2 AC 1.

3:8   Refusal of treatment

Competent adult patients have a clear right to refuse treatment for reasons which are "rational, irrational or for no reason".[12] In such cases, a health professional should explore the patient's reasons for refusal, correct any misunderstanding, and advise the patient of the increased risks of non-treatment and, if appropriate, other treatment options. No pressure should be brought to bear, but the patient should be allowed time to consider the information.

In some cases, refusal of the treatment recommended by a health professional may indicate that the carer-patient relationship has broken down and the patient may require a transfer to another health professional. If this is not the case, health professionals should not give the impression of abandoning the patient who has refused a specific treatment.

Where a patient's capacity is in question, it is important to give careful and detailed consideration to the patient's competency to make such a decision. It may not be the simple case of the patient having no capacity, but a more difficult case of a temporarily reduced capacity. Doctors should consider whether a person has capacity which is commensurate with the gravity of the decision which is to be made. The more serious the decision, the greater the capacity required. If the patient has the requisite capacity, then health professionals are bound by that decision. If not, they are free to treat the patient in what they believe to be his or her best interests. In cases of uncertainty, health professionals should seek a declaration from the courts as to the lawfulness of treatment.

If it is believed that the patient's prior views were opposed to life-prolonging treatment, health professionals should seek substantial evidence of this before considering curtailment of treatment. Such evidence may be in the form of an advance statement or "living will".

3:9   Refusal of basic care

3:9.1   Competent people

Basic care can be refused by a person who understands the implications of so doing. Basic care is defined as assisting people to do those things which they would normally do for themselves if they were able, such as keeping themselves clean, warm, dry and comfortable. There is a long established legal principle that every person's body is inviolate. Legally, therefore, competent people can object not only to medical treatment, but to any form of physical contact. It is the person's consent which renders physical contact lawful. For example, if a competent person refuses to accept food, it would be both unethical and illegal to forcibly feed that person.[13]

Carers should attempt to discover why the person is declining care. Ascertain whether the refusal represents, for example, a protest or need for attention or is symptomatic of the onset of a depressive illness which could be treated. You should attempt to persuade the person to accept care if failure to do so would lead to deterioration of his or her health or would present a health hazard to other people.

In residential institutions, in particular, there may be a conflict between the interests of a resident and the interests of the community in which he or she is living. While domestic routines and rules are necessary for the smooth running of residential institutions, they should not be so strict that they unreasonably restrain the residents' freedom to make their own decisions about their lifestyle. Like any other people, older people for their own valid reasons may refuse to get out of bed, eat meals at set times or wash on request. Generally, such objections are unlikely to have any serious consequences and may be accommodated.

If   a   resident's   behaviour   endangers   or   seriously

inconveniences others, then some action by staff is necessary. Initially, positive encouragement should be the first option, and the individual's attention should be drawn to the problems their behaviour causes for themselves and for others. Gentle persuasion or coaxing may eventually encourage the person to agree to change his or her behaviour, or to consent to (or at least not refuse) assistance from carers. If the resident cannot be managed in this way, expert advice should be sought from other disciplines; a community psychiatric nurse, for example.

A house officer in a rehabilitation unit for older people requested a consultant psychiatrist to see Mr Jones, who had suffered a stroke, was very disturbed, aggressive, unmanageable and violent towards the nurses. The psychiatrist was not available, so the nurse manager requested a psychiatric nurse specialist to visit the unit.

On visiting the unit, it was established that the patient's wife, Mrs Jones, was filing a formal complaint about his care. Mr Jones was aggressive, but examination of the environmental factors revealed that he was being nursed in a room on his own, and was being given too many different instructions. He was not being given time to make decisions and choices within his limited cognitive ability. Mrs Jones had not had a chance to express her fears of loss of her husband to a nursing home, and the psychiatric nurse sat with the wife for half an hour listening and enabling her to off-load her feelings of despair.

With some management and guidance, the nurses were able to cope with Mr Jones and his wife withdrew her formal complaint.

Close liaison between health professionals and psychiatric health professionals is essential, because some mental health problems may be caused by an undiagnosed physical problem.

George Lane is in his late eighties, is physically disabled, is suffering with dementia, and lives in a residential home. Mr Lane was becoming more disturbed, and the home owner asked the community psychiatric nurse (CPN) to visit as she thought he needed more Melleril to curb his aggressive outbursts. The CPN conducted a nursing assessment and discovered that Mr Lane's catheter bag was empty. On further questioning of the staff, the nurse discovered that Mr Lane had not passed any urine that day. The nurse concluded that he was in retention of urine. A bladder wash out was undertaken, and Mr Lane became less disturbed and didn't need any more Melleril.

3:9.2 *People who have fluctuating capacity*

Use the opportunities when the person is lucid to ascertain his or her wishes regarding care. Problems may arise if an older person has fluctuating capacity or is of borderline capacity. As a general principle, individuals need only demonstrate minimal capacity in order to consent to care which appears reasonable, non-invasive and in the interests of their welfare. They should, however, be able to demonstrate a more complete grasp of the implications in order to refuse care when that decision is likely to put their health and well-being at risk. This is not to say that they cannot make such a decision, but simply that their capacity to understand and retain what is at stake may require some form of verification before it is acted upon. For further discussion of this topic, see the BMA and Law Society's guidance on assessment of capacity.

Be cautious about taking advantage of a person's confused periods to provide care which had previously been refused while the person was lucid. Assess the value or the need of treatment in relation to the risk to the patient; do not simply accept the person's first response or automatically insist on giving care. If treatment is considered to be necessary, as a first step, try to encourage the patient to agree to the procedure in question. If negotiation with the patient fails, consider using other methods to gain the patient's cooperation. These need not be demeaning to the patient, but instead might use the patient's confusion in a constructive way to persuade him or her to accept a procedure which is to the patient's benefit. (See also chapter 2.)

Mr Ashton, a confused elderly man, is incontinent and refusing to take a bath. He will not only be at risk of developing pressure sores but his actions will also affect other patient's comfort in the ward. In order to offer preventive care and ensure others' comfort, a nurse may feel he or she has an obligation to bathe Mr Ashton. The nurse might give him a chance to make decisions, within boundaries. For example, he or she might run the bath and tell Mr Ashton that it is ready for him, then ask whether he usually has bubble-bath or not. In these types of situations, the care given should extend only to that which is necessary either for the immediate health care needs of the patient or those of other patients on the ward.

3:9.3 People who are incapacitated

When a person is considered unable to consent or refuse basic care, any reasonable action in the best interests of the person would be justifiable.[14] In our discussions, we have supported the recommendation of the Law Commission:

Anyone who has care of an incapacitated person (or has reasonable grounds for believing a person in his or her care to be incapacitated) may do what is reasonable in all the circumstances to care for that person and to safeguard and promote his or her welfare.[15]

We conclude that the provision of care is essential when the individual cannot consent. We also consider that basic care should not be rejected in advance by an advance statement or by a person appointed by the patient to make decisions on their behalf, although any form of treatment can be refused by an informed and specific advance statement.

Difficulties may arise particularly when someone who is incapacitated is actively resisting care which is in his or her best interests. Ways to deal with such problems are best illustrated through the following case examples.

Mr Stephens, a previously fit, older man, lived alone and had no relatives or neighbours who kept in touch with him. He presented to his GP acutely confused and doubly incontinent as a result of a chest infection, but he declined admission to hospital, treatment or care. Initially, his GP tried to encourage him to agree to go in to hospital, but when this failed the GP approached a local geriatrician and asked him to make a home visit to persuade Mr Stephens to receive treatment at home. In this situation, Mr Stephens agreed.

Mr Shah is an older man who was previously reasonably well and independent. He was admitted to hospital with an acute confusional state. Examination revealed that he was pyrexial and initial investigations revealed blood and protein in the urine, suggesting he had a urinary tract infection. Mr Shah was disorientated and aggressive. He repeatedly hit the attendant medical and nursing staff, stating that he did not want any treatment and that there was nothing wrong with him.

- **Step one:** Assess the patient's capacity with respect to the relevant medical decision.

- **Step two:** If the patient is judged incompetent, a decision on treatment should be made in his or her interests, and medical and nursing staff should attempt to persuade the patient to accept such treatment.

In considering the case, it was concluded that Mr Shah *did not have capacity* to make decisions with respect to his treatment and that it was in his best interests that his urinary infection be treated with intravenous antibiotics. The doctor attempted to persuade him to have the antibiotics, but failed.

- **Step three:** If the patient refuses treatment, and if time permits, environmental changes should be made to calm and reassure the patient, and further attempts made to persuade him or her to have treatment.

Mr Shah was taken from the noise and bustle of the main accident and emergency department to a quiet room where he was offered a cup of tea by a nurse who also attempted to persuade him that it would be best for him to receive intravenous antibiotics. This too failed to convince him.

- **Step four:** If time permits, a friend or relative should be contacted to try to persuade the patient to have treatment.

Mr Shah's son was contacted and tried to convince his father that it would be best if he received antibiotics. Despite this, he continued to refuse treatment but agreed to come into hospital. A decision was made to allow him to think about things for a few hours in the hope that he would agree to treatment.

- **Step five:** As a last resort, the patient could be sedated and treated.

After transfer to the ward, Mr Shah became more aggressive and confused. As all other methods had failed, he was sedated and given the antibiotics.

Eighty-year-old Miss Smith wanted to discharge herself from hospital believing that she would be able to look after herself at home. She had a non-dominant hemisphere parietal lobe infarct with major visual and spatial defects, yet denied she had any difficulties with day-to-day activities such as bathing and mobility. Miss Smith believed "things would be all right" once she got home, that she would not require help, and that she wanted to be discharged that very day.

Risk assessment showed what Miss Smith could and could not do at home on her own, and the medical team explained to her the difficulties she would have looking after herself. The team then enlisted the help of people Miss Smith trusted, including the nurses who had particularly been responsible for her care and the occupational therapist who showed Miss Smith some of the problems she would face if she were at home on her own. At the same time, relatives were asked to help persuade Miss Smith that it would be best for her to stay in hospital a little longer. Finally, it was agreed that Miss Smith should visit home for a day, or perhaps a weekend, with the occupational therapist to see how she managed. This experiment was repeated several times so Miss Smith had a good idea of what it would be like to be at home alone.

If Miss Smith was still sure that she could manage, she would be doing so in full knowledge of the facts.

3:10   The National Assistance Act

If older people are not looking after themselves at home, or not being looked after properly by carers, public health physicians have compulsory powers under section 47 of the National Assistance Act 1948 and an emergency procedure under the 1951 Amendment, to transfer people to a residential care facility. Much seems to depend on local circumstances, since the provision is used infrequently and very variably throughout the country, and is thought by some to carry some kind of stigma.

As with the right to refuse treatment, people have the right to live in squalor and to neglect or deny themselves personal care (the Diogenes Syndrome). Problems arise when these actions create a downward spiral so that the person becomes incapable of personal care, constitutes a danger to others, or when carers feel they can no longer work in such unsatisfactory conditions. In such cases the question of competence is often raised, but action under the Mental Health Act is rarely appropriate.

The public health physician must be satisfied that the conditions are insanitary, that the person cannot be provided with appropriate care in the existing situation, or that there is a danger to others (eg, risk of gas explosion). The evidence must then be brought before a Magistrate's Court or, in an emergency, a single magistrate, before the patient can be confined for periods of up to three months or three weeks respectively. Compulsory powers relate only to removal and the provision of care. There is no provision for compulsory treatment.

If an incompetent patient falls within the remit of the Mental Health Act, they may be removed from home.

3:11 Advance statements

It is essential to ensure patients are fully informed before creating an advance statement. People who know or suspect that their mental faculties will deteriorate in the future can make advance provision for later decisions. Advance statements ("living wills") provide a mechanism whereby competent people give instructions about what they would wish to be done for them if they lose the capacity to decide such matters. The most common use of advance statements is to register an individual's views about particular medical treatments, particularly life-prolonging treatments. Advance statements that apply to future medical treatment or non-treatment should be drawn up only when people are fully informed of the implications of their decisions. Dialogue between patients and health professionals is therefore essential.

3:11.1 The legal position

Presently, there is no specific statute to clarify the extent to which health professionals are legally bound by advance statements. Certainly, advance statements that authorise certain procedures or convey general impressions regarding preferences cannot be seen as legally binding, although a *clear refusal* of specific procedures may be. Nevertheless, it is clear that general statements of preferences should command respect just as any other expression of a patient's views.

In *common law*, a person who is fully informed and understands the implications of the decision, can make an anticipatory refusal of treatment which would legally bind health professionals if the decision were applicable to the circumstances which subsequently arose.[16] The statement must be unambiguous and must clarify the specific treatments rejected. A clear and informed statement refusing blood by a Jehovah's Witness is an example of a potentially legally binding document.

People with some forms of mental disorder or who are subject to delusions can also make a valid and legally binding (at common law) advance statement as long as they are clear about the consequences of the particular decision they wish to make.

In the 1993 case of "C"[17], a man in his sixties, who was confined to Broadmoor, suffered from the delusion that he was medically qualified. C refused amputation of a gangrenous foot and his anticipatory decision to continue to reject such an operation in future was upheld at law. C suffered from a mental disorder, but was considered competent to make the particular decision in question and to ensure that his current views would be upheld in future when his mental capacity might further deteriorate.

The BMA has published a code of practice for health-care professionals on the use of advance statements.

3:12   Cardiopulmonary resuscitation and do-not-resuscitate orders

It is unethical not to seek the patient's views regarding CPR or DNR if he or she is capable of expressing an opinion and resuscitation could be successful. Cardiopulmonary resuscitation may present particular ethical dilemmas for health professionals. Who should be involved in discussions about do-not-resuscitate decisions? Health professionals, patients and relatives have conflicting views. Although the literature on this subject encourages discussion with patients, in practice many doctors do not believe patients should be involved in DNR decisions and do not tend to consult them.[18] By contrast, patients and relatives believe they should be involved in discussions about CPR. Although many health professionals may find it difficult to raise the issue with patients, experience indicates that if it is discussed in a sensitive and realistic manner by an appropriately trained person at a suitable time, patients are not necessarily made anxious by the topic.[19] For further discussion, see the BMA and

RCN joint statement published in 1993, *Decisions Relating to Cardiopulmonary Resuscitation.*

Relatives should be consulted about DNR *only* with the patient's consent (if he or she is competent). Health professionals often find it easier to talk to relatives than patients about resuscitation decisions, and indeed relatives may want their "loved ones" excluded from such discussions. However, the patient's views *must* be sought (if he or she is capable of expressing an opinion) unless either it is felt that discussion would harm the patient in some way, or that resuscitation would be futile. It is also important to remember that a patient may not wish relatives to be a party to DNR discussions.

If the patient is not competent, health professionals should make resuscitation decisions on the basis of what is in the patient's best interests (see section 3:5). In such circumstances, those close to the patient should be consulted in order to ascertain what the patient's wishes would have been had he or she been able to make a decision.

It is important to consult all relevant members of the medical and nursing team about DNR decisions, as their perspectives may help in reaching a final decision. There should not be a policy of automatically excluding groups of people from resuscitation purely on the grounds of age. Decisions must be made on an individual basis. The entire health care team should be informed if a DNR order is made and the decision must be noted in both the medical and nursing records. Lack of awareness among the team of a DNR order can result in inappropriate resuscitation of a person and distressing prolongation of life.

3:13   Consent to research

Researchers, health professionals and local research ethics committees that approve research protocols should try to ensure that any agreement to participate in research (especially involving an entire group of residents or patients) represents the free choice of each individual. It is important to encourage research in diseases and conditions which affect older people. Studies aimed to benefit the older population often cannot be carried out adequately on other age groups since reactions or metabolism rate, for example, may vary with age. In addition, some diseases which particularly affect older people, such as Alzheimer's disease, have been shown to have a genetic component and it is possible that people suffering from it will want to participate in research which may ultimately benefit other members of their family even if it cannot benefit them. This is known as non-therapeutic research.

It is important to provide adequate advice and information, in accessible language, to enable older people to make a valid, independent decision. Older people have the same rights as all other adults to consent or to refuse to participate in research projects. However, people who are hospitalised, residing in an institution, or who otherwise feel themselves to be in a situation of dependency, may feel under pressure to conform with the wishes of others. It is therefore essential that they are given the opportunity to consent freely to participate in research and that they know that they can withdraw their consent at any time.

If a person is incapacitated, the 1990 case of *Re F* established the principle that necessary treatment in the person's best interests would be authorised. Therapeutic research, such as a randomised control trial looking at the effect of a promising therapy which is designed to benefit that person, is likely to be permissible but, like all research, should be submitted to the scrutiny of a local research ethics committee (LREC). Ethics committees seem to have difficulty in permitting research involving complementary therapies, but we encourage them to approach such research with an open mind.

Nurses were undertaking a development project using aromatherapy to determine if clients with dementia, who did not respond to orthodox methods of night sedation, would be helped by massage using aromatherapy oils. The development project was submitted to the ethics committee who decided that the project could not be done with people in dementia, because they could not give their informed consent about the use of aromatherapy oils.

The lawfulness of non-therapeutic research which involves physical contact with the incapacitated person, however, is more doubtful. Some bodies, for example the Medical Research Council, argue the case for non-therapeutic research involving only minimal risk if, it benefits people in the same category, cannot be carried out on other consenting sections of the population and if the incapacitated person gives no indication of objecting.

We consider that non-therapeutic research which directly involves an incapacitated subject is ethical if:

- the research cannot effectively be done on people who have the capacity to consent; and
- the research entails only an insubstantial foreseeable risk to the subject's physical or mental health; and
- the research has local research ethics committee approval; and
- the current, or past, wishes of the patient have been obtained if it is possible to do so;
- if not, the purpose of the research, the procedure to be used, and the foreseeable risk to the participants have been explained to those close to the patient; and
- the subject does not object, or appear to object, in either words or action to participating in the research, and has made no anticipatory decision refusing to participate.

Although there is no legal basis for substituted judgements, from an ethical point of view we feel that they could be made if it was known that the person would have wished to participate in research projects which would be likely to benefit either medical research generally or members of his or her family in particular.

3:14   The legal liability of treatment and care providers

Treatment given to a competent person without his or her valid consent may be considered battery in law. The subject of the treatment does not have to prove that he or she suffered harm from the procedure merely to demonstrate that it was non-consensual. Unauthorised touching, for example, is considered to be sufficient harm even if it is to save the person's life or health.

Overriding a competent person's refusal of treatment would be regarded by the courts as equally or more serious. A clear and specific refusal expressed through an advance directive could have the same force. A Canadian doctor[20] who saved the life of an unconscious Jehovah's Witness, but by means prohibited in a card the patient was carrying, was subsequently found guilty of assault. English courts[21] have expressed the view that the same conclusion would be reached in this country.

Although the 1990 case of *Re F* established that a doctor can lawfully treat an incapacitated patient provided such treatment is in the patient's best interests, it is not always clear to health professionals whether they have legal authority to proceed with treatment which is necessary, particularly if it has serious implications. Thus, we feel there may be value in health professionals being given *statutory authority* to carry out treatment which is reasonable in all the circumstances in order to safeguard and promote the best interests of the incapacitated person (or a person whom he or she has reasonable grounds for believing to be incapacitated). The statutory authority, however, should not permit the carrying out of any treatment which the incapacitated person refused by way of an advance statement.

10 Department of Health, Welsh Office. 1993. Code of Practice, Mental Health Act 1983. London: Department of Health.
11 The law on treatment of incapacitated patients was clarified in 1989 by the case of Re F [1990] 2 AC 1.
12 Per Lord Templeman in Sidaway v Board of Governors of the Bethlem Royal Hospital and Maudsley Hospital [1985] AC 871 at 904, 1 All ER 643.
13 It has been agreed by the Law Commission, and other bodies, that although competent individuals can refuse basic care currently, they should not be able to do so through an advance directive. Nor should a proxy decision-maker be entitled to refuse basic care on behalf of an incapacitated person.
14 Lord Goff in the case of Re F [1990] 2 AC 1.
15 English Law Commission. 1993. Mentally Incapacitated Adults and Decision-Making: A New Jurisdiction. London: English Law Commission.
16 Re T [1992] 4 All ER 649.
17 Re C [1994] 1 All ER (819–825).
18 Hill ME et al. 1994. Views of Elderly Patients and their Relatives on Cardiopulmonary Resuscitation. BMJ 308: 1667.
20 Malette v Shulman 1990 67 DLR (4th) 321 (Ont CA).
21 Re R [1992] 4 All ER 649, and Re C [1994] 1 All ER.

Chapter 4
Consent and
Confidentiality

Health professionals are responsible to patients for the confidentiality and security of any information obtained during the course of their work. There must be no use or disclosure of any confidential information gained in the course of professional work for any purpose other than the clinical care of the person to whom it relates, unless the person has given explicit consent to its disclosure. However, there are exceptions to this rule. Those most relevant to the care of older people are:

- disclosure of information between health professionals, on a need-to-know basis, for the care of individual
- rarely, when it is in the clinical interests of the patient to inform relatives and other carers, and it is impossible or undesirable to seek the patient's consent
- rarely, when disclosure is in the public interest or in the interests of the individual.

Each of these will be discussed in further detail in the following sections. For further discussion of situations in which it is acceptable to disclose information without consent, see the BMA's publication *Medical Ethics Today, its practice and philosophy.*

4:1   Sharing on a need-to-know basis

It can generally be assumed that patients have given *implied* consent to the sharing of health information with other health professionals who need to know the information in order to provide health care to that person. However, as health care is increasingly being provided in multi-disciplinary teams, it is important that people are made aware of this and encouraged to be actively involved in decisions about when and to whom information should be disclosed. A written statement setting out the general guidelines which govern the sharing of information may assist these decisions.

4:1.1 Multi-agency liaison

Inform clients explicitly of the circumstances in which information about them is likely to be shared, so that they can take part in decisions about which personnel should be involved in their care. The implementation of the NHS and Community Care Act 1990 has encouraged a shift in emphasis from professional decision-making to the active involvement of individuals and their carers. This has fostered a culture of "empowerment" where provision of services is based on the needs and desires of clients and their carers. The encouragement of multi-agency and multi-professional assessment and planning of care packages embodies working in partnership with clients, and offering a range of service provision options from various public and independent service providers.

An older person's consent to disclosure within the multi-agency team should not be assumed, even on a need-to-know basis and that person's case notes should not be made readily available to everyone in the team. Cohesive and cooperative working arrangements among all service providers need to be in place if a variety of agencies and individuals are to participate fully and actively in decision-making about aspects of care that will enable older people to remain at home. With the patient's agreement, only the information that is *necessary* for a particular member of the team to carry out his or her duties effectively should be revealed to that person. Sharing identifiable information for the convenience or interests of health workers or administrators is not acceptable.

4:2 Liaising with relatives and other carers

4:2.1 When it is impossible or undesirable to seek a person's consent

Disclose to carers only as much information as is necessary to care for the patient properly and only if

there is no reason to believe that the patient would object.
This should be applied in those rare situations when it is
considered to be in the patient's clinical interest to disclose
information to carers or relatives so that they can help manage the
patient's condition, but it is either impossible or clinically
undesirable to seek the person's consent.

When people with dementia are living in the community, it is
possible that the only carer is a neighbour. In order for the person
to manage alone, confidence may have to be broken so that
appropriate care can be delivered.

For example, Mrs Hillier, an older woman, lives in a warden-
controlled flat but the warden worries about her. The community
psychiatric nurse (CPN) may have to talk to the warden about Mrs
Hillier's behaviour, indicating what to look out for that could be
considered a risk, and how to respond in these circumstances. In
this way, the warden will be informed enough to reduce her own
anxiety and to allow Mrs Hillier to continue to live alone without
unnecessary interruption. The relationship between Mrs Hillier,
the CPN and the warden can be crucial in preventing unnecessary
alarm or anxiety and may help prevent Mrs Hillier's premature
admission to hospital.

4:2.2   Social security "special rules" for people who are dying

The government has instituted "special rules" procedures for
people who are terminally ill and thought to have less than six
months to live. In some cases, the patient will not wish to know the
full prognosis, but carers may need financial assistance for his or her
care. Information can be passed from the patient's general medical
practitioner to another doctor employed to assess the patient's
need, without the patient necessarily being aware of this exchange
of information. If the patient is not the initiator of the benefit
application, carers are inevitably involved and safeguards are in
place to minimise the risk of inadvertent disclosure to those who
may not wish to know (ie, the patient) or do not *need* to know for the
purposes of care.

4:2.3   When the patient can be consulted

When a patient can be consulted there is a delicate balance to
achieve between allowing the individual to decide who is told what,

and when, about the condition and appropriate care and treatment, and not making relatives or other carers feel excluded. Be prepared at least to listen and talk to the relative or carer, although it will be a matter of judgement what information you should disclose in return, bearing in mind the patient's wishes about confidentiality and the disclosure of information.

An example of where the balance went wrong involved a consultant and the son-in-law of an older woman. The consultant refused to speak to the son-in-law without the woman's written permission, when the son-in-law simply wanted to tell the consultant that his mother-in-law was convinced she had cancer because the consultant had requested a radioisotope study.

If older people are able to express their wishes, take time to consult them properly or to identify the particular factors which are reducing their ability to communicate and help them overcome such difficulties. In the case of very ill patients or older people who are hard of hearing or have difficulty communicating, there may be a tendency to discuss the patient's care primarily with relatives simply because it is quicker and easier. In some cases (for example when the patient is unable to retain information), this may be the only solution. In others, however, a patient may not have the means to communicate easily. In these situations patients should be helped to express their views by being given appropriate aids, such as hearing aids or communicators. Simply taking the patient to a quiet room where there is less distraction may also help the patient express what he or she wants. Patients also may respond better to the approaches of particular staff or relatives.

Mrs Ward, an anxious 80-year-old woman, was admitted to hospital following a stroke causing a moderately severe hemiplegia and dysphasia. A decision had to be made as to whether she should return to her own flat or should move into residential care. Both Mrs Ward's daughter and the speech therapist spent long periods of time trying to elicit her views on this matter. The process was, however, hampered by the fact that Mrs Ward appeared to become much more anxious in the presence of either her daughter or the speech therapist. Mrs Ward did, however, communicate well with a particular staff nurse on the ward, whom she knew and trusted, and it was through this channel that her wishes became clear.

4:2.5 *Using interpreters*

Use an interpreter if the patient does not know English, speaks poor English, speaks with a strong accent, or has difficulty understanding the accent of a health professional. In these situations, there may also be a tendency to discuss a patient's care with carers and relatives. Be cautious, however, about automatically involving a relative as an interpreter. While relatives may be more easily accessible than independent interpreters, and the patient may be reassured by the presence of some one familiar, some patients may not want a relative to hear sensitive or intimate details and may prefer an unknown and impartial interpreter to be involved in the consultation. Furthermore, relatives may unwittingly (or otherwise) put their own interpretation on the information, which may unduly influence a patient's decisions.

4:2.5 *Nominating a representative*

With the older person's agreement, it may be helpful to nominate one relative to liaise with the health team and impart news to other family members. When many relatives are interested in the care of a patient, such as the children of an older person, they may all try to be involved in discussions about the management of their parent's care and may give conflicting views. Nominating one spokesperson helps avoid confusion for all concerned.

4:2.6 *Using citizen advocates*

Because of confidentiality considerations, exercise some caution when involving citizen advocates fully in discussions about the patient's care. Citizen advocates are trained volunteers who act on behalf of people who may have difficulty representing their own interests. They can be invaluable in helping a patient to express his or her views if there are difficulties in communication. As the advocates are neither a relative nor associated with the health care facility, they can offer assistance without being influenced by conflicting interests. It is important to establish clearly on whose authority the advocate is acting. If an older person has sought the advocate's support, then the extent of their involvement will be guided by the wishes of that person. Difficulties may arise for the health care team when an older person, who is either incompetent or has fluctuating competence, is newly admitted to hospital or some other facility and an unknown person is presented as the person's advocate. In such situations, the team may not know whether the person is self-appointed or, indeed, representing the patient at his or her request and therefore will be uncertain as to how much the advocate should be included in discussions about care and how much his or her views should be heard. If there is any doubt, then the duty of confidentiality to the patient should prevail until the precise status of the advocate is confirmed.

In order not to undermine the valuable contribution advocates can make in defending a vulnerable person's interests, it is important that their role is clearly defined and that mutual understanding and cooperation is fostered between advocates, the health care team and the patients involved. Presently, citizen advocacy projects are established locally on an ad hoc basis, although there are a number of national organisations which offer advice, support and training to local initiatives. The Centre for Policy on Ageing has developed a code of practice for citizen advocacy with older people aimed at people involved in the management and operation of advocacy projects. To ensure the highest standards of training and practice, we recommend, in addition, that a recognised registering and disciplinary body be established to monitor and regulate practice in this area.

4:2.7 *Maintaining confidentiality in hospitals or residential facilities*

All health care staff have an obligation to respect the privacy of residents. Care should be taken not to talk freely between each other about residents, nor in earshot of other clients. People of any age who spend long periods in hospital or institutions often report losing their sense of self-identity. Frequently, it seems that when there is bad news to be given about the patient's prognosis, the patient may be the last person to know. Most people are able to decide for themselves whether they want to know the full details of their condition or prognosis, whether they prefer to have only a general idea, or if they prefer not be told at all. The decision cannot be made for them by other people, but the cues regarding information and confidentiality should come from the patients themselves.

Keep records containing personal health and other information securely, and limit access to those with overall responsibility for the day-to-day care of a resident. The provisions of the Access to Health Records Act 1990 apply equally to residents in hospital or other facilities as to all other patients. For written guidance on this Act, contact the Ethics Department at the BMA.

4:3 Disclosure in the public interest

If disclosure is felt to be necessary in the public interest, health professionals must take care to ensure that the information is disclosed only to appropriate personnel or agencies and not communicated haphazardly. Exceptionally, disclosure without consent may be justified when it is in the public interest or in the interests of an individual. This situation might occur when the failure to disclose appropriate information would expose the patient, or someone else, to a risk of death or serious harm, or when the person is a risk to public health because he or she is suffering from a serious infectious disease and refuses to take precautions to prevent others being infected.

The British Medical Association has received reports, for example, of patients' HIV status being widely divulged to other staff and residents in residential facilities when the risk of infection to these people was almost non-existent. While health professionals clearly have an obligation to ensure the safety of other residents and carers, routinely disclosing such information to residents is not likely to achieve anything except the alienation of those labelled as a risk. Instead, it is important to give careful thought to establishing routine preventive measures against infection for all residents and to channelling resources into training staff in safe practices and routine precautions. Obviously, health professionals have to take decisions to share information in some circumstances, but they should always have clear grounds for disclosure and a good idea of what they expect the recipient to do with the information revealed.

4:3.1 Fitness to drive

Health professionals should raise the issue of ability to drive when they know that a person suffers from a visual

impairment or medical condition which makes driving hazardous. Driving despite deterioration in their ability to do so (due to failing eyesight or other conditions) is a common situation in which older people may constitute a risk to themselves and the public. Currently, there are no standard procedures for assessing older people's competence to drive. The DVLA does not request a driver to undergo a medical examination unless it has received a report questioning the driver's ability. It requires drivers over the age of 70 to indicate that they consider themselves fit to drive, but there is no requirement that this statement be supported by medical opinion.

If there is disagreement or uncertainty as to the extent of the patient's impairment, health professionals should draw to the person's attention the importance of obtaining an objective view from a driving examiner. Individuals with suspected impairment can obtain independent evaluation of their driving skills at specialised driving assessment centres.

After informing the patient of the danger of driving, actively encourage the patient to inform the licensing authorities and indicate that you will do so if the person continues to drive. This may require further follow-up. Doctors should ask the person to return after considering the matter and inform them of the action they have taken. Patients should be aware that withdrawal of licence is not necessarily automatic, since options exist for a second medical opinion and an independent assessment of competence to drive. In exceptional circumstances, health professionals may consider breaching confidentiality in the public interest, but before doing so they should tell the person of their intention.

4:4 Confidentiality and the abuse of older people

There is no system for the obligatory reporting of the abuse of a vulnerable person in this country and care must be taken not to breach confidentiality. A dilemma arises for health professionals when they suspect that a person living in an institution is being abused, but the victim refuses to allow the situation to be reported. This may be for fear of the abuse worsening or out of a sense of loyalty, guilt or responsibility.

The dilemma may take two forms. In some situations the only source of information about the abuse is the patient. In this situation it is difficult to report the abuse without the patient's consent. In other cases, there may also be observable signs or evidence of abuse, making it easier to report independently of the victim's consent. The situation is made more difficult in an institutional or family setting where others may potentially be at risk of abuse. It may take some time for an older person to come to a decision about revealing abuse and he or she should be offered counselling and support to assist in the decision.

We recommend that education about elder abuse should form an integral part of the undergraduate and post-graduate curricula for health and caring professions. Abuse of older people is generally poorly understood by health professionals. Organisations such as Action on Elder Abuse are currently working to bring this issue to the attention of health professionals and the public, and to provide guidelines in this area (see Further Reading). It is imperative that this work reaches health professionals early in their careers.

Chapter 5
Consent and the Use of Protective Measures

5:1 Using protective measures

Protective measures may be needed to control restless or agitated behaviour which might endanger the older person or others if it continues unchecked. This can be achieved in many ways, using simple and obvious means; not least by treating the older person as an individual with his or her own needs and wants in what may seem to be a strange and unsympathetic environment.
Protective measures may include:

- Spending time talking to the person, whether or not he or she appears to understand, and encouraging the person to talk about things that may be bothering him or her. Thoroughly explain the reasons for routines and actions in the hospital or residential facility to the person.
- Allowing people to expend pent-up energy by giving them space to move around freely. Do not place furniture in ways which will obstruct their movement. In addition, give people the opportunity to spend some time outside in fresh air.
- For demented patients who wander, lay out the environment in such a way that the patient can wander freely, either inside or in the garden, yet always return to the point of departure. In this way, patients can go for a proper walk, with variety, on their own, while staff can be assured of their safety.

- Arranging activities which will keep older people interested and occupied. Boredom can be a cause of restlessness and disruptive activity.
- Placing the mattress of restless patients on the floor or lowering the bed, rather than using cot sides. Bear in mind that restlessness may occur because the client is wet, needs to go to the toilet, is thirsty, hungry or too hot or cold.
- Providing suitable exercise and other activity, or complementary therapies (such as massage), which may help relax clients[22], rather than using sedatives or other medication.
- Encouraging friends and relatives to visit frequently, as this can be a calming influence on confused and restless older people.

5:1.1 Use of photographs

There is an ethical dilemma in keeping photographs of vulnerable clients on file. The photo can be used to search for the person if he or she wanders. While it might be useful to have a photograph of a client who is particularly vulnerable and likely to wander, this person is least likely to be able to consent to having the photograph taken. In exceptional circumstances, however, having a photo of a patient on file may be in the best interests of the patient as a way of ensuring his or her safety.

5:2 Use of restraints

In broad terms, restraint means restricting someone's behaviour to prevent harm, either to the person being restrained, or to other people (the Royal College of Nursing and other agencies have published a comprehensive range of literature on issues of seclusion, control, and restraint which are listed in the Further Reading section). Restraint should be used only for a short duration and only as a final resort, when all other measures for preventing harm have been exhausted. Methods often used for restraining people, which vary in acceptability, include harnesses, cot sides, sedative drugs and arranging furniture to impede movement. Cot sides, for example, are generally avoided because it is felt that the harm caused by falling from the greater height imposed by the cot side does not justify any benefit derived from restraining the patient. Restraint is not only physical; it could involve, for example, carers wrongfully using their authority to dissuade a person from leaving a room.

It is important to make clear the reasons why a particular form of restraint is considered to be necessary in a given situation. Although the use of restraints in exceptional circumstances may be necessary, there is a fine line between the use and abuse of restraining measures. The most routine procedure, for example, catheterisation, or a seemingly innocent arrangement of the furniture could be seen as unacceptable restraint in some circumstances. Use of restraints should be discussed by the whole health care team, fully documented, and reviewed regularly.

5:2.1 *General principles for using restraints*

When considering the use of restraints, keep these principles in mind.

- The purpose of restraints should be to allow people the maximum amount of freedom and privacy compatible with their own safety.
- The method used should always be the minimum possible in the circumstances, and should be used only for as long as is necessary to end, or reduce significantly, the threat to the patient or to other people.
- Competent adults who may need such measures, but who do not endanger others, must understand the purpose and give consent. Older people may wish to accept certain risks in order to enjoy greater freedom of movement, and health professionals should be careful not to overprotect individuals by unduly restricting their activities. Staff should make a balanced judgement between the need to promote an individual's autonomy by allowing him or her to move around at will, and the duty to protect the person from likely harm.
- Where any form of restraint is proposed to protect mentally incapacitated people from hurting themselves, restraint should be used only to the extent of preventing risk beyond that which would normally be taken by a similarly frail, mentally alert person.
- Restraint should **not** be used simply to aid the smooth running of the health care facility, or as a substitute for sufficient staff. Nor should it be used as a punishment. A gross abuse of the use

of restraints came to public attention in late 1992 when a mentally handicapped woman died in hospital after being tied to a lavatory cistern by a bib and left for 45 minutes while staff had their lunch.

Mr Roberts has dementia, is having reminiscences about the war and believes he has to escape from the Germans. The staff discover him trying to climb out of the window on the first floor. The nurses are unable to persuade him to climb down from the window and they finally have to physically restrain him and bring him back in.

In another situation, Mr Chester, who is demented, believes a lady is his wife (although she is not) and he is very protective towards her. When her husband visits, Mr Chester becomes very aggressive towards him. Because he is unable to comprehend the true situation and cannot be encouraged to calm down, the nurses have to remove him physically from the lounge.

In these and similar situations, issues and procedures to consider are:

- Is the person at risk of his or her actions, either immediately or in the longer term?

- Are others at risk from the patient's behaviour?

- If yes to either of these points, can the person be persuaded to change his or her behaviour?

- If the danger to the patient or others is not imminent, health professionals could consider withdrawing for a while to allow the situation to cool down before trying again.

- If this does not work, and it is imperative that the person is prevented from doing something, then the health professionals should consider whether there are any other preventive measures that could be employed.

When all options have been exhausted, restraining measures may be necessary and justifiable.

5:2.2 Unintentional restraint

Nursing and medical staff should be continually observant for unintentional restraints, as older patients often do not question their loss of mobility, accepting it as an inevitable consequence of hospitalisation. Not uncommonly, older people are unintentionally restrained following a transfer from one environment to another. For example, an elderly patient admitted to hospital may be accidentally deprived of his or her walking stick and thus be unable to walk, might be seated on a chair which is too low and therefore be unable to stand, or might be catheterised but not given a leg bag, and so unable to move around.

5:2.3 *Seclusion*

As with any form of restraint, seclusion should be used only as a last resort where all reasonable steps have been taken to avoid its use. Seclusion is defined as the "supervised confinement of a patient alone in a room which may be locked for the protection of others from significant harm".[23] It should not be used if there is a risk that the patient may deliberately harm him or herself while in seclusion, if there are staff shortages, or if there is a risk of damage to property.

The use of seclusion to protect older people, who would be at risk of harm if they were allowed to wander out of a ward or nursing home at will, should be discouraged. Instead, such people should be protected by improved surveillance provided by an appropriate number of staff. Alternatively, the use of electronic tagging devices may be helpful means of giving older people greater freedom, while giving protection at the same time (see section 5:3.1).

5:3   Other preventive measures

Older people who have dementia and who are prone to wandering outside the home or health care facility, are a significant cause of anxiety for health professionals and other carers. Locking doors of wards and other rooms may be one way of preventing older people from wandering, but this measure is subject to a certain amount of criticism. Health professionals often feel there is some justification in locking rooms, because it provides a safe area in which patients may wander freely. Within this area, the risk has been assessed and staff are generally comfortable in accepting the risk involved. Outside this area, concerns for patients' safety become serious. However, locked doors may also restrain others who have no reason to be restrained and we question whether it is right that the freedom of these people should be restricted in order to protect the few who wander.

Two alternative measures to protect wandering patients are currently the subject of debate: 1) the use of removable electronic tagging devices to track those who wander, and 2) boundary crossing alarms which alert carers when the patient strays beyond a certain distance or past an alarmed door. Some people believe both measures are degrading and dehumanising.[24] If used appropriately, we believe that both can be helpful.

5:3.1 Removable electronic tagging devices

The use of removable electronic tagging devices should be used only as a last resort and should not be used as an alternative to supervision by an adequate number of staff. The use of devices which are be surgically implanted under the skin cannot be justified. Removable tags can be beneficial to people with dementia by allowing them greater freedom and safety, thus enhancing their liberty. They can also help carers by providing reassurance. The use of tagging devices can enhance both safety and liberty, because they enable residents to be found more quickly and also enable carers to offer a less restrictive form of care. Tagging should not be used as a substitute for adequate care by staff, but should be used to complement staff efforts. Health care staff cannot be expected to watch constantly for wandering patients. Such intense monitoring would diminish attention given to other residents and would limit the staff's ability to carry out other equally important duties.

Despite the potential benefits of electronic tagging, it can be abused. Electronic tags should be worn only with the consent of the person involved, if he or she is capable of making this decision. Many residents for whom tags will be proposed will not have such capacity; therefore, decisions to use them must depend upon whether it is in the best interests of the patient. It is important also to involve those close to the patient in discussions, so they can be reassured that the use of tagging is strictly necessary.

Before introducing tagging devices in practice, a Code of Practice should be drawn up outlining the circumstances in which they may be used. Their use should be monitored and audited.

5:3.2 Boundary alarms

We agree with the view expressed by McShane et al[25] that if a locked door is justified, then a boundary crossing alarm must also be justified because the restriction of the wandering person's liberty is the same. Use of alarms may be preferable to locked doors, because they do not restrict the liberty of other people.

5:4 Developing policies for use of restraints

All institutions should have policies for the use of restraints. The policies should identify good practice and outline proper procedures for monitoring and reviewing the type and frequency of restraints used. Alternatives to the use of restraints should be identified and encouraged. Staff should also identify where restraints are used due to inadequate staffing or other resources, and should bring this to the attention of the health authority or health board.

22 Royal College of Nursing. 1992. *Focus on Restraint*, ed 2. London: RCN.

23 Royal College of Nursing. 1993. *Seclusion*. London: RCN.

24 Counsel and Care. 1993. *People not Parcels: a discussion document to explore the issues surrounding the use of electronic tagging on older people in residential and nursing homes.* London: Counsel and Care.

25 McShane R, Hope A, Wilkinson J. 1994. Tracking Patients who Wander: Ethics and Technology. Lancet, 343: 1274.

26 English Law Commission. 1993. Mentally Incapacitated Adults and Decision-Making: A New Jurisdiction. Consultation paper no. 128. London: English Law Commission.

27 English Law Commission. 1993. Medical Treatment and Research. Consultation paper no. 129. London: English Law Commission.

Chapter 6
Conclusions and Recommendations

Health professionals and others involved in the provision of health care for older people face numerous challenges. This report has considered those raised in connection with the ethical and legal principles of consent which guide medical and nursing practice. The practical guidelines and suggestions offered below represent standards of good practice.

General

1. Older people have the same rights to services and health care as any other members of society. Health professionals, therefore, have an obligation to ensure that the rights of older people are not eroded in the provision of health care. As with all individuals, access to care and treatment should be decided on the basis of clinical need and ability to benefit, not on the basis of age.

Consent

2. Health professionals must seek the views of all patients, whenever possible, concerning their care and treatment. Although some older people might have difficulty communicating, hearing or understanding, this does not lessen health

professionals' obligation to consult older patients and to gain their consent to care and treatment programmes.

3. Health professionals should provide comprehensive, understandable information **prior to** seeking a patient's consent and **during** treatment, so the patient can decide whether to request the treatment to be altered or stopped.

4. When people are not able to consent to care and treatment, through reasons of incapacity, health professionals must give the care and treatment that is necessary to promote the patient's health and well-being. The consent of the next-of-kin is not needed and is not recognised in law. Nevertheless, it is important to involve those close to the patient in decisions (if they are available) as they might be helpful in indicating what the patient would have wanted, if the patient had been competent to decide.

Refusal of treatment

5. Competent adults have a clear right to refuse treatment for any reason.

6. Health professionals should explore the patient's reasons for refusing treatment in case there might be any misunderstanding. They should also advise the patient of the risks of non-treatment and, if appropriate, other treatment options.

7. We support the principle of advance statements. These enable people to specify how they would like to be treated if they lose the capacity to decide or to communicate.

8. In common law, an advance statement made by a fully competent person is legally binding on health professionals if the decision applies to the circumstances which subsequently arise.

Refusal of care

9. Competent people have a right to refuse basic care. Carers should attempt to discover the reason behind the refusal, as it may reveal certain needs which are not being met by the health care team.

10. Attempts should be made to persuade the person to accept care if the failure to receive care would lead to a deterioration in the person's health, or the health of other people.

11. We consider that patients should not be able to reject basic care (to keep them clean, warm, dry and comfortable) in an advance statement, nor should a person acting on the patient's behalf be able to refuse care

12. Although certain domestic routines and rules are necessary to ensure the smooth running of residential institutions, these should not be so strict that they unreasonably restrain the residents' freedom to make their own decision about their lifestyle. Residents' wishes should be accommodated as long as they do not seriously inconvenience or upset others.

Do-not-resuscitate orders

13. With sensitive issues, such as do-not-resuscitate orders, it is tempting to speak to an older person's family rather than to involve the patient in possibly distressing discussions. If patients are competent to take part in such discussions their views must be sought unless: (a) resuscitation would be futile, (b) discussion might harm the patient, or (c) the patient makes clear, either implicitly or explicitly, that he or she does not want to participate in such discussions, and nominates a proxy to be involved instead. Health professionals should take the cues from the patients themselves and should not make assumptions about their wishes.

14. Sometimes health professionals' reluctance to talk to patients about these issues is due more to their own discomfiture than the patients'. The education of health professionals increasingly includes training in communication skills, a move which we commend. However, we recommend that greater emphasis should be placed on training health professionals to communicate sensitively and effectively about issues concerning death and dying, with particular regard to older people. When discussing do-not-resuscitate decisions all relevant members of the medical and nursing team should be consulted, and the decision should be recorded in the medical and nursing notes.

Research

15. We believe that non-therapeutic research on an incapacitated patient is ethical if: (a) the research is into a condition suffered

by the subject, (b) it involves minimal risk to the patient (c) it has appropriate research ethics committee approval, and (d) the patient does not appear to object, in either action or words, and has made no anticipatory decision indicating a refusal to participate. Those close to the patient should also be consulted to ascertain what the patient would want, if he or she were able to consent.

Confidentiality

16. Older people have the same right to confidentiality as other individuals.
17. As a general principle, health professionals must seek the consent of a competent patient to the disclosure of personal information. Exceptions to this rule are described in the text.
18. When competent patients have difficulty communicating, health professionals must take time to try to understand the patient's wishes and should provide any aids and support that might assist in this process.
19. When a patient is incompetent, information should be disclosed only to individuals who need to have the information for the care and treatment of the patient.
20. In health care facilities, health professionals should ensure that records containing personal health and other information should be kept securely, with access limited to those with overall responsibility for the day-to-day care of residents.
21. Issues concerning the abuse of older people are poorly understood by health professionals. We commend the work undertaken by organisations such as Action on Elder Abuse to draw the issues to the attention of the health professions and the public. We believe that such work also needs to reach health professionals early in their careers; we therefore recommend that education about elder abuse should form an integral part of the undergraduate and postgraduate curricula of both medicine and nursing.

Citizen advocates

22. We support the role of citizen advocates in representing the interests of people who have difficulty in representing themselves. However, to ensure mutual understanding and

cooperation between advocates and health professionals, it is essential that the advocate's function is properly defined. We therefore commend the Centre for Policy on Ageing's initiative to develop a code of practice for citizen advocacy with older people, but further recommend the establishment of a recognised registering and disciplinary body to monitor and regulate practice in this area.

Restraints

23. Restraints should be used only when all other forms of controlling restless or agitated patients (who endanger themselves or others) have failed.
24. The entire health care team should discuss and record the use of restraints, and this record should be reviewed regularly.
25. Nursing and medical staff should be continually alert to situations where patients are unintentionally restrained, particularly following a transfer from one environment to another.
26. Restraints should never be used simply for the convenience of the health care team or as a substitute for inadequate staffing.
27. We believe the use of removable electronic tagging devices is ethical if its purpose is to provide greater freedom and safety to the individual concerned. However, before tagging is introduced, we recommend there be further research into its benefits and that a code of practice should be developed to regulate its use.
28. We recommend all institutions to develop formal policies for the use of restraints and other measures to protect the safety of individuals and others. These should outline proper procedures for monitoring and reviewing the type and frequency of restraints used. Alternatives to the use of restraints should be identified and encouraged.
29. Staff should identify where restraints are used due to inadequate staffing or other resources and should bring this to the attention of the health authority. Furthermore, we consider that both doctors and nurses have an obligation to report serious abuses of the use of restraints to the facility's management, and where appropriate the General Medical Council or United Kingdom Central Council for Nursing,

Midwifery and Health Visiting, and in doing so they should have the full support of their respective professional bodies.

30. In addition to the statutory inspection of residential facilities, which is infrequent, we recommend that local authorities should establish procedures whereby local authority officers can visit regularly any residential and nursing home without notice, to inspect the facilities.

Glossary

Basic care: measures that help people (sick or well) perform activities contributing to health, which he or she would do unaided given the necessary strength, will or knowledge. It includes the provision of both paid and unpaid, formal and informal, services by health professionals, commercial enterprises, families and others to people who are unable to accomplish for themselves what they would like to do. Care includes assisting a person to meet requirements for food, drink, contact, warmth, personal hygiene and protection from injury.

Best interests: Much of this report refers to people who need various types of assistance and support but are mentally competent to decide issues for themselves. The concept of judgements being made on a "best interests" basis applies only to mentally incapacitated people who need decisions to be made for them. We have adopted the Law Commission's definitions of the criteria for a "best interests" judgement in relation to (a) care and (b) treatment.[26, 27]

(a) Care
(1) the ascertainable past and present wishes and feelings of the incapacitated person;
(2) the need to encourage and permit the incapacitated person to participate in any decision-making to the fullest extent of which he or she is capable;
(3) the general principle that the course least restrictive of the

incapacitated person's freedom of decision and action is likely to be in his or her best interests.

(b) Treatment

(1) the ascertainable past and present wishes and feelings (considered in the light of his or her understanding at the time) of the incapacitated person;

(2) whether there is an alternative to the proposed treatment, and in particular whether there is an alternative which is more conservative or which is less intrusive or restrictive;

(3) the factors which the incapacitated person might be expected to consider if able to do so, including the likely effect of the person's life expectancy, health, happiness, freedom and dignity.

Health care decision: surrounding major decisions about whether to accept or refuse particular aspects of care, diagnosis or treatment, there will be many smaller decisions which lead to it. People who are judged incapable of making valid, major decisions may still give a valid response to a lesser matter and should be consulted. The contrary may also be true. A person may be capable of deciding on a major matter, such as whether or not to undergo mastectomy or amputation, but may be less able to understand the implications of lesser interventions, such as preventive measures.

Incapacity: mental impairment which prevents an individual from understanding the nature and effect of the particular decision which needs to be made, or from retaining information long enough to make a choice. Capacity can only be assessed in the context of the activity which is to be decided. Thus, the fact that a person lacks capacity to make a will or a contract, does not necessarily mean he or she lacks capacity to make valid decisions about medical treatment. (See BMA and Law Society guidance on the assessment of capacity). The presence of mental disorder may not mean that an individual is incapacitated.

Medical treatment: includes all forms of medical intervention. It includes pain relief, as well as artificial nutrition and hydration for people who are unable to swallow sustenance put into the mouth.

People may have particular anxieties about pain, especially the likelihood of terminal pain. Pain relief is a medical treatment rather than a facet of basic care. It is the fundamental right of every person to have access to appropriate and adequate pain relief (whenever this is attainable). Health professionals have an ethical obligation to ensure that they know how to obtain information about specialist pain relieving techniques. Competent people, if properly informed, have the right, currently, to refuse any medical treatment, including pain relief. They may decide to do so, for example, if it is important to them to retain as much lucidity as possible to interact with family and friends. We consider it unwise, however, for competent people to try to decide upon limitation of future pain relief through an advance statement. Nor should a proxy decision-maker be able to limit the pain relief accorded to an incapacitated person, even if previously nominated by that individual to make medical treatment decisions. The precise role and powers of a proxy decision-maker have not yet been defined in law.

Substituted judgement: the "substituted judgement" test is sometimes used as an alternative to the principle of "best interests". Under this test decisions regarding care and treatment of an incapacitated person are judged on the basis of what the person would have chosen if he or she had been competent to decide, rather than on what a health professional or proxy considers to be best for that person. This test requires the subjective values of the individual to be taken into account insofar as they can be known.

Useful Addresses

Action on Elder Abuse
Astral House
1268 London Road
London SW16 4ER
0181 679 8000

Age Concern England
(as above)

Alzheimer's Disease Society
Gordon House
10 Greencoat Place
London SW1 1PH
0171 306 0606

British Association for Service to
the Elderly
119 Hassell Street
Newcastle Under Lyme
Staffordshire ST5 1AX
01782 661033

British Federation of Care Home
Proprietors
852 Melton Road
Thurmaston
Leicester
LE4 8BN
0116 264 0095

British Medical Association
BMA House
Tavistock Square
London WC1H 9JP
0171 387 4499

Centre for Policy on Ageing
25-31 Ironmonger Row
London EC1V 3QP
0171 253 1787

Help the Aged
16-18 St James Walk
London EC1R OBE
0171 253 0253

Law Commission
37-38 John Street
Theobalds Road
London WC1N 2BQ
0171 453 1220

Law Society
113 Chancery Lane
London WC2A 1PL
0171 242 1222

National Care Homes Association
5 Bloomsbury Place
London WC1A 2QA
0171 436 1871

Registered Nursing Home Asso-
ciation
Calthorpe House
Hagley Road
Edgbaston
Birmingham B16 8QY
0121 454 2511

Relatives Association
5 Tavistock Place
London WC1H 9SS
0171 916 6055

Royal College of Nursing
20 Cavendish Square
London W1M 0AB
0171 409 3333

Further Reading

A scandal waiting to happen, RCN, 1992

An inspector calls? the regulation of private nursing homes and hospitals, RCN, 1994

Bill governing the use and disclosure of personal health information, BMA, 1995

Briefing pack, Action on Elder Abuse, 1994

Citizen advocacy with older people; a code of good practice, Centre for Policy on Ageing, 1994

Code of practice for health professionals on advance statements, BMA, 1995

Decisions relating to cardiopulmonary resuscitation, BMA and RCN, 1993

Focus on restraint, ed 2, RCN, 1992

Guidelines for doctors and lawyers on assessment of mental capacity, BMA and Law Society, 1995

Medical Ethics Today, its practice and philosophy, BMA, 1993

Mental Health Act Code of Practice, chapter 18, HMSO, 1993

Mental Incapacity. Summary of Recommendations, Law Commission report 231, HMSO, 1995

Mentally incapacitated adults and decision making, medical treatment and research, Law Commission document 129, HMSO, 1993

Rights and Responsibilities of Doctors, BMA, 1992

Seclusion, RCN, 1993

Seclusion, control and restraint, RCN, 1992

The privacy of clients, electronic tagging and closed circuit television, RCN, 1994

What if they hurt themselves, Counsel and Care, 1992

Index